T0154378

Kindness...
Is The
New Cool

Susan Elizabeth Clark

Kindness... is the new cool

How to open doors, melt
hearts & make everyone happy

OH EDITIONS

Kindness:

It costs nothing — and means everything!

Anon

Introduction

In *Kindness Is The New Cool* we'll be celebrating all the good things that can (and will) enter your life once you decide to make Kindness your daily practice and the currency of your choice. I'll show you how to keep Kindness top of your daily 'To Do' list and how to practice kindness until it becomes second nature to you.

There are some fun and easy exercises which help us to become even kinder and even more compassionate; and if you work your way through these and build Loving Kindness into the fabric of your everyday life, you'll discover too how kindness bounces — just like a happy boomerang — out from you to others and, before you know it, right back to you.

This is the little book that reminds us there is a currency available to us all that opens doors, melts hearts and makes everyone touched by it happier.

Plus, it's a choice!

You can be kind, or you can be mean but if you choose the latter, you'll be missing out on the New Cool that is Kindness with a capital 'K'.

It's become cool to talk about Random Acts of Kindness, but Kindness is a profoundly spiritual gift and life choice and so 'random' doesn't cut it.

We don't need random acts — we need all our actions to be based on a new, Radical and deeply profound version of Kindness that runs through our core and shows up in everything we think and do.

As if we had no other choice.

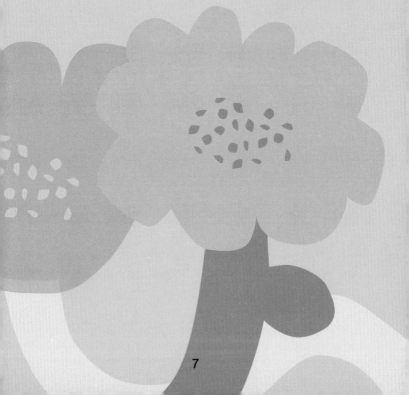

8

In the
Kindness Store
Cupboard

The ingredients you'll need to get started on becoming kinder:

An open mind

An open heart

A new journal (dedicated solely to learning about and practising Kindness)

Colouring pencils and drawing paper

A small candle or tea light (for the yogic practice of candle gazing to focus your mind on Kindness)

A yoga or other non-slip fitness mat (to practice some simple and safe poses that help open the heart chakra — your body's loving-energy centre)

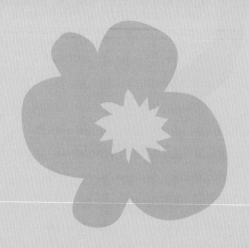

Kindness is a gift every single
one of us can afford to give.

Unknown

Kindness is a language which the blind can see and the deaf can hear.

African proverb

11

CHAPTER ONE

Kindness Opens Hearts and Doors

Kindness will open doors for you to realise your dreams, and for others to realise theirs too. Remember, confident and successful people don't need to tear others down to stay that way. There's plenty of room for everyone, so if you can make an extra space for someone else and do them the kindness of giving them a boost or a lift up then do so. You'll be amazed how quickly that act of kindness comes back your way opening unexpected door for you, paying unimagined dividends and more.

But before we can use Kindness to open hearts and doors, we must learn to be kinder and more compassionate with a capital 'C' to ourselves.

Be kinder to yourself.
And then let your
Kindness flood
the world.

Pema Chadran
BUDDHIST NUN AND TEACHER

EXERCISE

List three kind things somebody's done
for you over the past month.

List three kind things you've done for
someone else over the past month.

Start each new day with a promise
to do one kind thing for yourself and one
kind thing for someone else. Every day. And
before you know it, you've got a new habit
and one that makes you (and others) happy!

Happily, learning to be kinder is fun and
will make you feel better about yourself.
So, open up your Kindness journal and
let's get started.

Why not text or call a friend you've not heard from in a while and check they're doing ok, or you could send flowers or a 'Thinking of You' card to someone you know is having a hard time.

And there's so many ways you can be kinder to yourself: from banishing that critical internal voice that's always trying to rubbish you; to making sure you're eating well and taking better care of yourself physically.

Showing Compassion and Kindness towards yourself (and others) will always make you feel good about yourself.

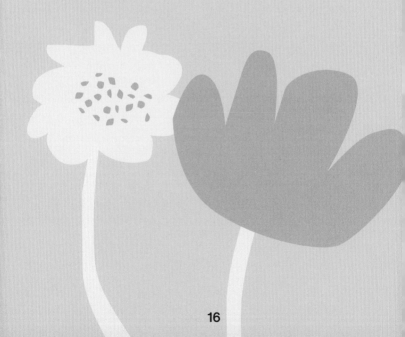

Kindness is a passport
that opens doors and
fashions friends.

It softens hearts and
molds relationships that
can last lifetimes.

Joseph B. Wirthlin
RELIGIOUS LEADER

Be Kind to Yourself

Kind acts shouldn't just be something we reserve for others. We should all be a lot kinder to ourselves and the first important step towards that goal is to forgive what's gone before.

You may have done things you're not proud of and don't want to think about. You may not have been as kind as you know you could have been to someone else and for that, you need to forgive yourself.

Perhaps thre was someone in your life who was unkind to you? They may have said or done something spiteful and hurt your feelings. Try to forgive them too.

When British TV actress, Jenna Coleman, was asked what she'd learned from the year 2020 that she would be taking into the year 2021, she said:

'We need to slow down. There's a feeling that you always need to be achieving something or pushing forward, everyone's diaries are choc-a-block, and we try and multitask on such a level that we forget the beauty of just surrendering.

I've appreciated the stillness, and also the kindness.

I feel like there was so much of that around at the beginning of lockdown.

I hope it continues.'

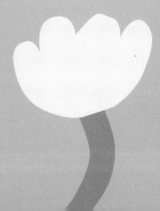

Forgiveness Mantra

A mantra is any word or phrase that
we repeat to bring our focus back to
a specific topic. You can say the words
out loud or in your head.

> I forgive what's
> already happened.
>
> Nobody can change
> that now.
>
> I forgive myself.
>
> And others.
>
> I'm starting over,
> and I'm doing that
> right now.

In your
Kindness journal

List three kind things
you've done for yourself this week.

List three kind things
you've thought about yourself this week.

Now, list three unkind things
you've done to yourself this week.

List three unkind things
you've thought about yourself this week.

Be as honest as you can
when you think about this.

Which list was the easiest to write?

I'm guessing you could probably fill an entire journal with a list of ways you've been mean and unkind to yourself.

It can be tempting to let Negative Self Talk run the narrative of our lives and if that is the case, you will be someone who could fill an entire journal with lists of the horrid things you've told yourself.

Negative Self Talk also batters our self-esteem and self confience so the sooner we can silence it – using kindness and kinder thoughts and feelings about ourselves – the better.

If I'm wrong about this, congratulations, you're already on the way to a well-deserved and well-earned Certificate of Kindness.

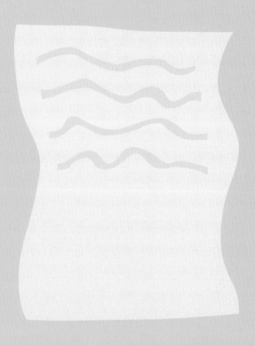

My wish for you is that you continue.
Continue to be who and how you are,
to astonish a mean world with your
acts of kindness.

Continue to allow humour
to lighten The burden of
your tender heart.

Maya Angelou
AUTHOR AND ACTIVIST

23

Radical Acts of Kindness Towards ... Guess Who? YOU!!!!!!

This will feel like it's your birthday and every other High Day and holiday celebrations rolled into one.

Because today is the day you start treating yourself with the same Kindness that you'd show to someone else. One easy way to make this positive change and start practising treating yourself with more kindness is to change the harsh tone of that voice inside your head and to push back when it starts being unkind towards you.

If you want to be clever about this, imagine this 'voice' belongs to someone who doesn't yet know how to behave around other people and that your job is to teach them kindness.

So, the next time the 'voice' says something mean to or about you just gently point out there is never any need for unkindness – especially towards yourself!

Kindness Planner

In your Kindness journal, write down
all seven days of the upcoming week.

Now, next to each day, write one thing
you will do that makes you happy, makes you feel
good about yourself and tells your inner critic to
butt out — because you've decided (from now on)
to be much kinder to yourself.

Stuck for ideas?
Here are some to inspire you:

Monday

home spa treat

Tuesday

coffee catch up with a mate

Wednesday

treat your body to a Buddha bowl lunch
packed with superfoods

Thursday

buy yourself flowers or a new houseplant

Friday

re-read a favourite poem or book

Saturday

take a trip to a favourite spot in nature,
cherish this time out

Sunday

pad about in your socks — all day!

To err on the side of kindness
is seldom an error.

Liz Armbruster
WRITER

Kind words are like keys.
If you choose them right,
they can open any heart
and shut any mouth.

Unknown

You only have control
of three things in your life;
the thoughts you think,
the images you visualise,
the actions you take.

Jack Canfield
AUTHOR AND MOTIVATIONAL SPEAKER

How Kindness Opens Doors

Kindness opens doors because people who cross paths with you will remember your actions — especially your radical and profoundly kind actions — long after they forget your words. And the more authentically and profoundly kind you become the more people will remember you.

Kindness, as we are seeing, is the New Cool. Being kind makes you cool and people always want to hang out with the cool crowd, whether that's at work or at play.

Your kindness will make a really good and lasting impression when people first start getting to know you.

Then, when an opportunity comes along, yours will be the name in the forefront of their mind.

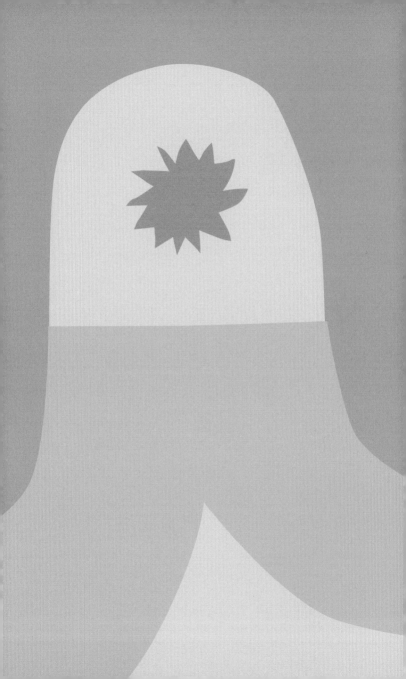

If our hearts are ready for anything, we will spontaneously reach out when others are hurting. Living in an ethical way can attune us to the pain and needs of others, but when our hearts are open and awake, we care instinctively.

Tara Brach

PSYCHOLOGIST, AUTHOR AND BUDDHIST

33

CHAPTER TWO

The Art of Kindness

Here are the best things about Kindness —
it is available to everybody, all of the time,
and it is absolutely FREE.

Imagine accidentally discovering one of the
best things in life – kindness – and realising not
only is it freely available to you, your supply will
never ever run out. You can use as much as you
like every day and when you come back, there's
always plenty more waiting for you.

Plus, it is contagious and, once released,
will happily run rampant.

Plant the seed
and watch it grow

Kindness starts with the self.
Kindness extends to the community.
Kindness embraces the whole world.

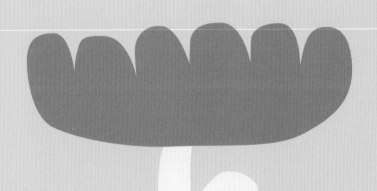

Now that I am old, I admire kind people. When I was young, I admired clever people.

Abraham Joshua Heschel
PHILOSOPHER AND THEOLOGIAN

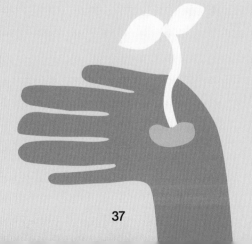

The Art of Kindness Starts with Acts of Kindness — Big or Small

You can cultivate mercy when you extend acts of compassion and kindness to yourself and to other people.

Bree Miller

MASTER BAKER AND INFLUENCER

The Lion and The Mouse

The lion was snoozing in the sunshine when he woke suddenly with a jolt. A tiny mouse had skittered across his nose.

The lion caught the offender as he tried to scamper away and after toying with him, thought about killing him.

But the terrified mouse pleaded for his life ...

'Let me live and one day, when I can, I will repay you.'

Now, if the lion had a fault, some said it was that he was too kind.

So, he let the little mouse go.

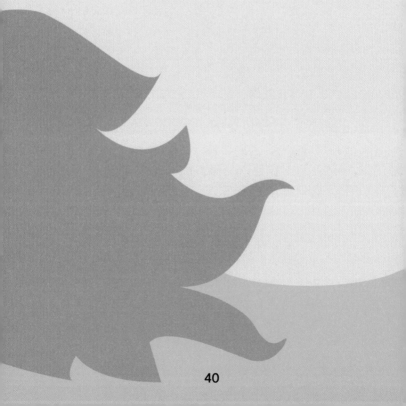

A few days later, the lion was hunting when he got tangled in a hunter's nets.

Unable to free himself, he roared with frustration and fury.

The tiny mouse recognised his voice and scurried to find out what was wrong.

Finding the lion enmeshed in the hunter's netting, she set about gnawing the ropes to free him.

The little mouse laughed as the lion shook himself free and told him: 'You laughed at me when I said one day I'd help you. But now you can see even a mouse can help a lion!'

This Aesop fable teaches us that even the smallest act of Kindness has meaning.

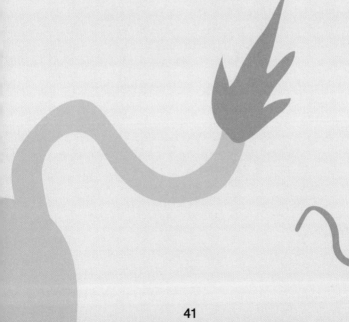

No act of kindness,
however small,
is ever wasted.

Aesop

Breathe Kindness In and Out

We can take this idea, of repeating a mantra to help us embody the Art of Kindness, a step further. Set aside just five minutes of quiet time every day to repeat a longer mantra.

Again, you can make up your own words but try and link them to the breath, like this one does, so that in time being kind is as natural and effortless to you as breathing in and breathing out.

Mantra

I can breathe in compassion

I can breathe out judgement

I can breathe in kindness

I can breathe out spite

I can breathe in peace

I can breathe out misery

Being mindful allows you
to think of others' situations and problems.
Walking by someone you don't know his or
her story, but you have the ability to be kind
and mindful of him or her.

Kellie Sullivan

ACTRESS

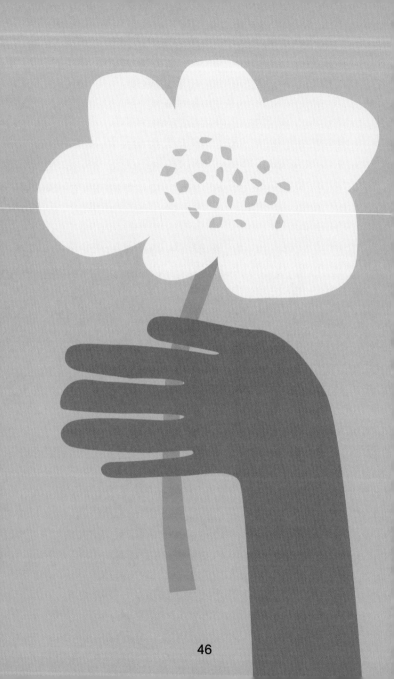

Use your voice for kindness,
your ears for compassion,
your hands for charity,
your mind for truth
and your heart for love.

Unknown

Kindness Symbols

A great way of bringing Kindness into
the heart of your home is to surround
yourself with symbols that remind you
Kindness is a choice. You can attach
a symbolic meaning to anything you
choose and even make your own
symbols but to help you get into that
way of thinking, here are some ideas ...

Take a large sheet of drawing paper
and colouring pencils from your Kindness Store
Cupboard and draw the outline of the biggest
heart you can.

As you draw, imagine all the Kindness that's ever
been shown to you filling this heart and when
you've done that, imagine all the Kindness you
show people piled on top of that.

Decorate your heart drawing
and pin it on the wall.

Say it with a Heart

The heart is the universal
symbol of Love that expands
out to include Kindness.

Say it with Flowers

Floriology — the use of flowers to convey a message or a meaning. In the Victorian Era, flowers held symbolic meanings. People sent coded messages to each other — of love and admiration and even admonishment — by simply sending a posy.

We may have lost this wonderful language of flowers from our culture today, but you don't have to dig too deep to find out what flower your Victorian ancestor would have known was a symbol of Kindness.

That flower is the humble but colourful Pansy.

As part of your new practice (of showing more Kindness and Compassion towards yourself) why not treat yourself to one if it is the right season; or make sure to buy seeds and grow your own when the time is right.

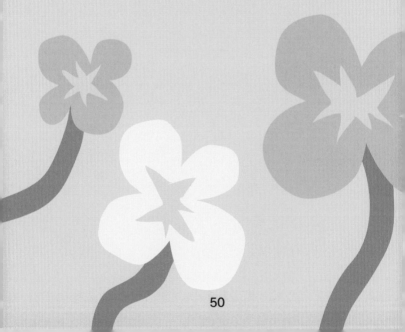

Elderflower is the plant that denotes Compassion in the secret language of flowers. Kindness and Compassion are intertwined, practice one and the other will naturally follow.

But don't try and put a sprig of elderflower in a posy as it will wilt in just a few hours after leaving the tree.

Instead, take a moment to admire an elderflower tree laden with blossoms and drink in their distinctive scent, thinking all the while of a wonderful life (yours) ruled by deep Compassion and great Kindness.

If you don't live in or near anywhere that elder grows, pop a bottle of elderflower syrup or juice in your bag next time you shop and when you pour it into your glass, take a moment before you enjoy the drink to breathe in the distinctive elderflower aroma.

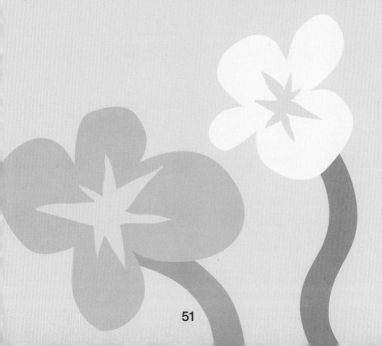

Say it with a Picture of a Deer

Esoteric traditions and indigenous cultures often attach
a symbolic meaning to animals, particularly the spirit of
that animal.

And the animal that is symbolic of Kindness is the deer.

Symbolising love, gentleness, kindness, grace and a shy
sensitivity, deer embody a purity of purpose. We can interpret
this purpose as our intent to be radically kind and deeply
compassionate to all souls — and of walking in the light.

Find a beautiful photograph or painting of a deer
and hang it on the wall.

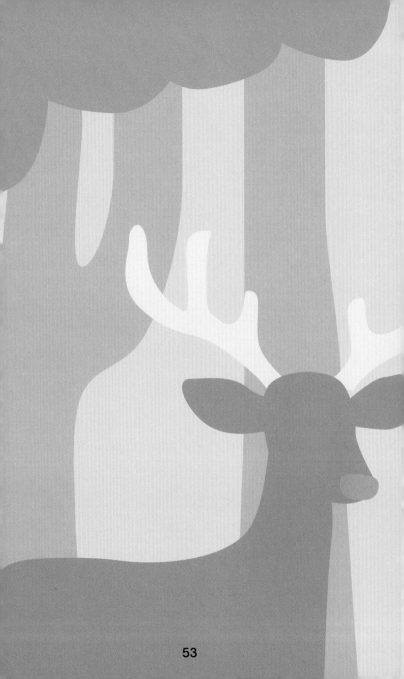

Say it with Colour

Pink is a calming colour that reminds us to be caring, nurturing, loving and, above all else, kind.

Wear something pink to remind you of the importance of Kindness and buy a rose quartz crystal to keep by your bedside.

Once cleansed*, your crystal will attract more Loving Kindness into your life and remind you when you wake each morning to practice being kind to yourself.

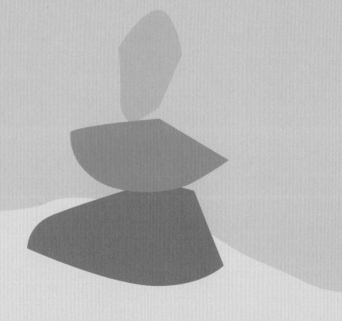

*Crystals absorb energy which is what makes them so useful in energy work, but this also means it is important to cleanse any crystal that is new to you and your home. We do this to make sure we are not susceptible to any energy it has already absorbed from others. You can cleanse your rose quartz by washing it with distilled water.

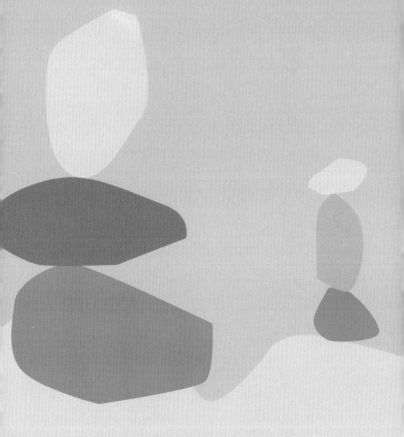

Less is more ... unless we're talking about kindness.

Unknown

Kind words are like keys
if you choose them right,
they can open any heart
and shut any mouth.

Unknown

Kindness is Free

So, sprinkle it both literally and metaphorically everywhere ...
If you like cinnamon on your morning coffee, think of
Kindness as you sprinkle. In fact, think of Kindness when you
add any spice to pep up the taste of a homemade dish.

Kindness is for Animals

Tuppence a bag ...

Remember the poignant song that Mary Poppins sings, when she and the children see an old woman in rags scratching out a living by selling bird seed to tourists in London's Trafalgar Square?

When you're throwing out bird seed for the birds, you are also engaging in a meaningful and profound act of Kindness.

In your journal, write down other kind things you can do for the wildlife you share your garden or patio or local park with; including picking up litter to prevent wild animals from harming themselves

If you're serious about showing Kindness to animals, then try doing these things:

Switch to cruelty-free beauty and lifestyle products.

Drop a food donation into the animal charity's collection box at the food store every time you shop.

Take your old towels and bedding to an animal shelter.

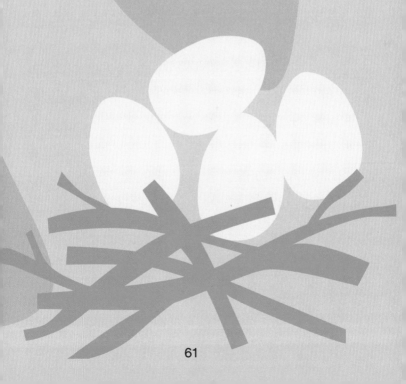

I can't prove it, but I think the reason we love our pets so much is because they remind us to always be kind. And when we remember to be kind, we feel better about ourselves and our lives.

So, the relationship really is a virtuous circle of Kindness.

Question:

How much pleasure do you get from feeding your cat or dog their favourite food? Watching them enjoy the freedom of a crazy run-around after a long morning cooped up indoors? Taking care of an elderly family pet who has shown you nothing but love and loyalty all their days?

We can learn much about the Art of Kindness from our family pets!

Proverb

The Battle of the Wolves

There is a battle of two wolves inside us all

One is evil. It is anger, jealousy, greed, resentment, lies, inferiority and ego.

One is good. It is joy, peace, love, hope, humility, kindness, empathy and truth.

The wolf that wins?

The one you feed.

Native American Indian proverb

I found it is the SMALL
everyday deeds of ORDINARY
folk that keeps the DARKNESS at bay ...
small acts of KINDNESS and Love

Gandalf — J. R. R. Tolkein
WRITER

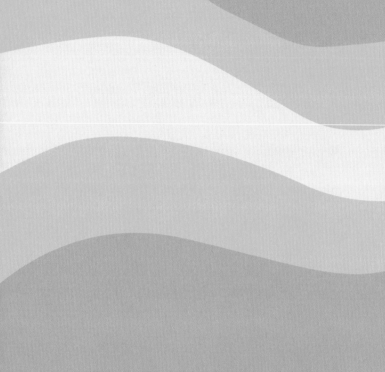

What we learn every time we read a tale of
Kindness or an inspirational quote is that the
Art of Kindness really is a choice.

We choose to be kind.

The trick is not only remembering this,
but also remembering to make this choice
each and every day.

Always pray to have
eyes that see the best,
a heart that forgives
the worst, a mind that
forgets the bad, and a soul
that never loses faith

Unknown

Kindness is seeing the best in others, even when they cannot see it in themselves.

RAKivist

WWW.RANDOMACTSOFKINDNESSORG

EXERCISE

1
Listen

2
Offer to help

3
Cook for someone, or just
make them a cup of tea

4
Hold someone's hand

5
Hold the door open

6
Smile at a stranger

7
Notice who is in the room
and say hello

Small Acts of Kindness

Too often we underestimate
the power of
a touch, a smile,
a kind word,
a listening ear,
an honest compliment,
or *the smallest act of caring*,
all of which have the
potential to turn a life around.

Leo Buscaglia
MOTIVATIONAL SPEAKER

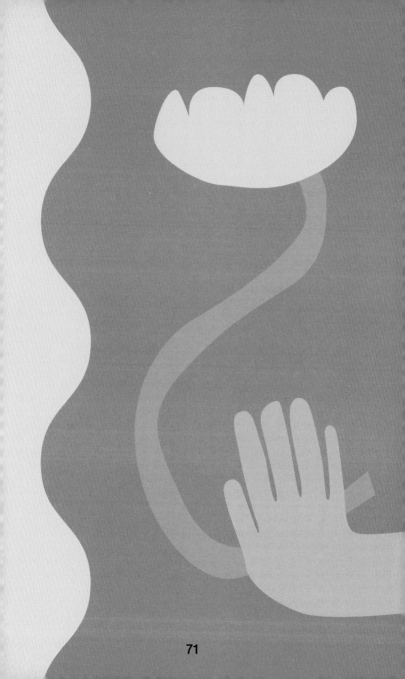

CHAPTER THREE

Kindness Melts Hearts

Kindness comes in many forms
but is always from the heart.

It also melts hearts.

And scientists now think being kind
is encoded in our DNA!

According to scientists who reported their
findings in the journal, Proceedings of the
National Academy of Sciences, being kind,
caring, empathic and trustworthy may be an
integral part of our genetical makeup and not
a genetic accident! How good is that?

Love and kindness
are never wasted.
They always make
a difference.
They bless the one
who receives them,
and they bless you,
the giver.

Barbara De Angelis
TRANSFORMATIONAL TEACHER

Melt Your Heart

It's impossible to separate love and Kindness —
one flows from the other and vice versa — so in
order to melt hearts, your own included, you need
to engage with your heart energy.

In order to do this, try this simple exercise:

Put your hand gently over your heart.

Close your eyes and *breathe slowly in,
to a count of five.

Hold your breath for another count of five and as you do so, imagine that all your power, all your love, all your efforts and all your goodness reside in the heart that is beating under your hand.

Now, as you exhale slowly to a count of 10, feel that strong connection to your heart energy and know you can come back to this loving place any time you like, just by repeating this exercise.

*Little tip: Try and get into the habit of breathing in and out through your nose and never through your mouth. This is a key yogi practice, you will never see a yoga guru breathe in or out of the mouth, and will help you better control the breath.

Kindness Heals
Deep Divides and Rifts

There's an old saying that goes something like this:

> 'You'll always catch more flies
> with honey than vinegar.'

It means you are more likely to persuade people to your point of view and change both hearts and minds with Kindness and softness than you are with bullying, aggression or control.

If you've had a falling out with anyone, either recently or in the past, think about the healing power of sending them a kind word, even an apology or a heartfelt admission of wrongdoing on your part.

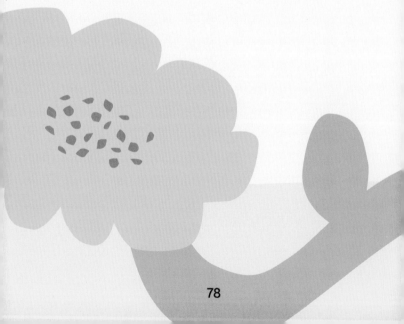

You could send a WhatsApp message saying you miss that person; or even go retro and send a notecard with a picture of something you know they like.

You don't have to believe me when I say choosing the path of Kindness can heal the deepest of rifts — try it for yourself and see.

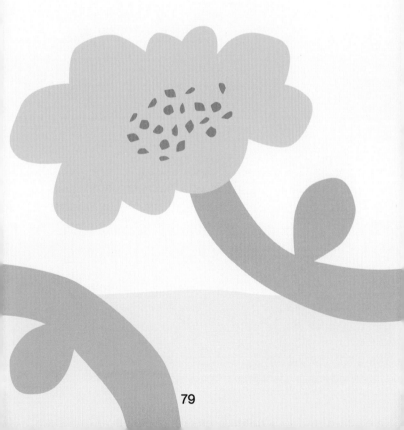

Profound Kindness

A lot of talk about Kindness focuses on the small kind and caring things we can do for each other.

Profound Kindness takes these steps further, until Kindness itself becomes the basis of our spiritual beliefs and practices — whatever their given name.

Kindness is not a new invention.

It has been an important part of spiritual beliefs for centuries; it may just feel like we've forgotten it because we've been ignoring it.

The antidote to all the division and the scepticism and the anger and the polarisation is to lead the way by living lives of profound kindness.

Dr Barry Corey
PRESIDENT, BIOLA UNIVERSITY

Kindness in the Christian Tradition

Kindness is no small thing. It yields marvellous fruit both in our lives and the lives of those around us.

Whoever pursues righteousness
and kindness will find life,
righteousness, and honour.

Proverbs, 21:21

Kindness in the Islamic Tradition

The Qur'an teaches us to be kind to people who are around us and show us that it really doesn't take much to be kind. Once you do it with a sincere heart and to seek the pleasure of Allah, an act of Kindness (al Ma'un) can turn into a reward to be counted on the Day of Judgment.

Prophet Muhammad says: 'Allah is kind, and He loves kindness in all matters.'

Kindness in the Jewish Tradition

'Chesed' is a Hebrew word that is often translated to mean Loving Kindness It is more than simply Kindness itself — it is super-powered Kindness. Many Jewish thinkers hold the value of Loving Kindness up as Judaism's primary ethical value and it appears more than 190 times in the Torah.

So central is the ideal of Loving Kindness to the Jewish faith, it is said that 'the beginning and end of the entire Torah is Loving Kindness.'

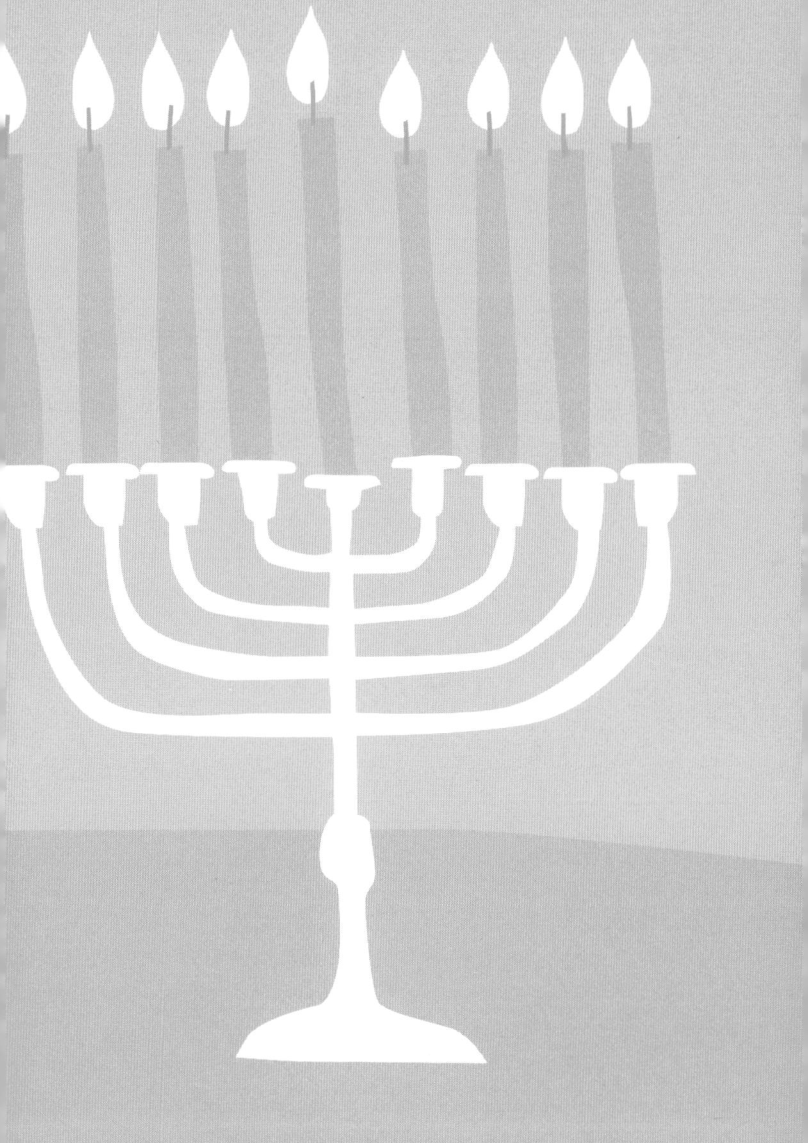

Kindness in the Buddhist Tradition

Profound Kindness is also central to the Buddhist Faith.
The quote below is attribued to Buddha himself:

'Our problems are not solved by physical force, by hatred,
by war. Our problems are solved by loving kindness, by
gentleness, by joy.'

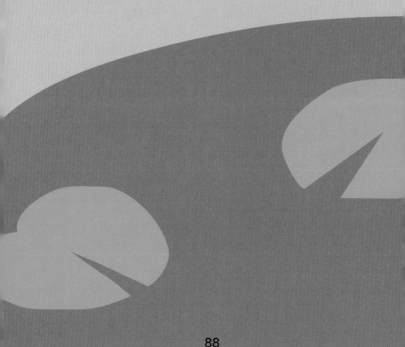

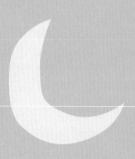

What wisdom can you find
that is greater than kindness?

Jean-Jacques Rousseau
PHILOSOPHER

Constant kindness can accomplish much. As the sun makes ice melt, so kindness causes misunderstanding, mistrust, and hostility to evaporate.

Albert Schweitzer
HUMANITARIAN

The great spiritual traditions make it clear that Kindness is not for nimbies. It is not about taking the easy way, to get your own way and it has nothing to do with being nice!

Being nice is all well and good but unlike Kindness (which requires us to make an effort and really connect with someone else) there's sometimes a more selfish agenda when someone is being unexpectedly nice — or nice to everyone, all of the time.

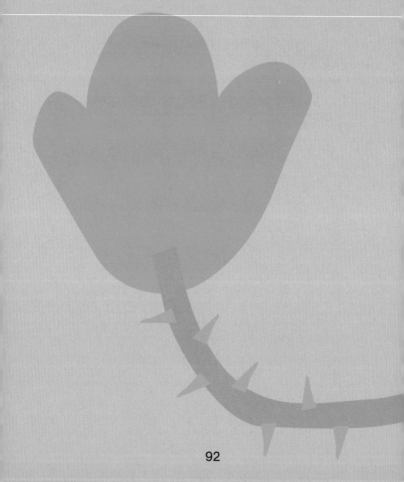

Profound Kindness asks us to dig a little deeper than that. And its biggest 'Ask' is that we show Kindness to all, in all our actions, no matter how badly we may feel we have been treated by someone.

I don't like you but ...

Take out your Kindness Journal and
a tea light candle for this exercise.

Write down the name of someone
you find it difficult to be nice to, let alone kind.
(This can be a family member, a work colleague,
a stranger who cut you up when driving, an
ex-lover or a neighbour who keeps dumping
stuff in your garden.)

Just make sure that whenever you think
of this person, you feel your whole body
tense with your dislike of them.

Now, light your candle and send one single kind thought toward this person.

You can say:

'I don't like you, but I can still send Loving Kindness towards you today.

My wish for you is that something lovely happens for you today.'

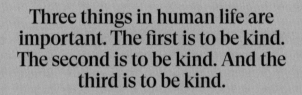

Three things in human life are important. The first is to be kind. The second is to be kind. And the third is to be kind.

Henry James
NOVELIST

Kindness is Strength

Don't mistake Kindness for weakness — it takes great strength of character and authenticity to stay kind when others are hurling (metaphorical) rocks and unjust accusations in your direction.

Stand firm in your Kindness. Do not be swayed.

Kindness always wins.

Do we want a world where all people are included? Do we want a world where all people have access to food/shelter/water/safety? If so, then this means looking Your opposition in the eye and allowing Yourself to say: 'You deserve food/shelter/water/safety too.' For this, we need daring diplomats. People who work to educate despite hate. (We can be compassionate without giving permission to someone to continue their actions.) We need many forms of existence all working towards the ultimate goal of unity. Many tools to grow a garden.

Rain Dove

MODEL, ACTOR AND ACTIVIST

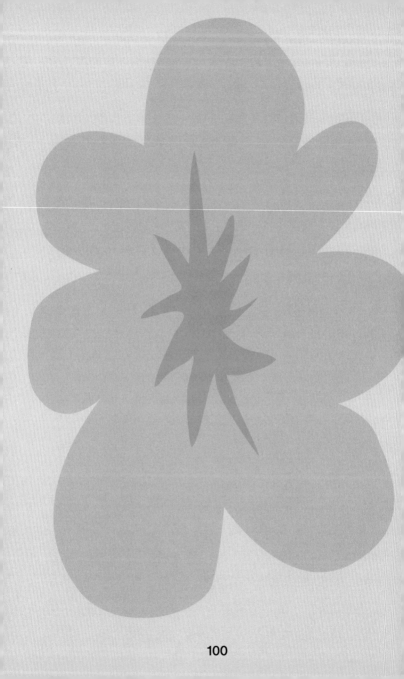

I have always felt that kindness

is love made visible.

Bronnie Ware
SONGWRITER AND AUTHOR

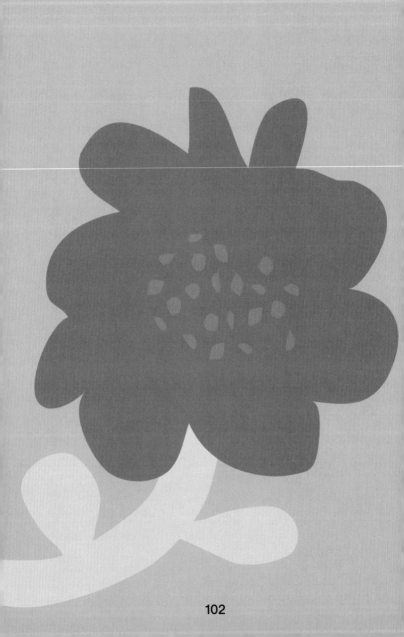

Kindness is the only service that will stand the storm of life and not wash out. It will wear well and be remembered long after the prism of politeness or the complexion of courtesy has faded away.

Abraham Lincoln
US PRESIDENT

A kind gesture
can reach a wound
that only compassion
can heal.

Steve Maraboli

BEHAVIOURAL SCIENTIST AND SPEAKER

The best and most beautiful
things in the world cannot be
seen or even touched they must
be felt with the heart.

Helen Keller
HUMANITARIAN

Cultivating Kindness

There are two definitions of the word 'cultivate' and if you think about it, they both apply to the practice of Kindness:

Cultivate
to prepare and use land for crops, or gardening.

Cultivate
to acquire, or develop, a quality or skill.

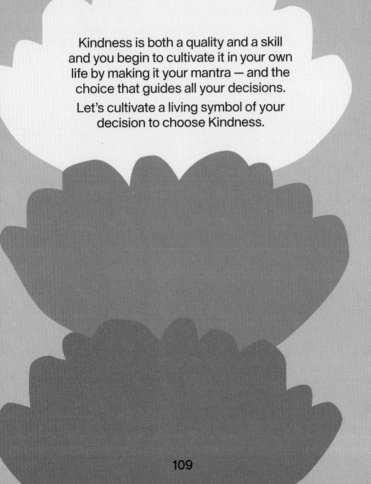

Kindness is both a quality and a skill and you begin to cultivate it in your own life by making it your mantra — and the choice that guides all your decisions.

Let's cultivate a living symbol of your decision to choose Kindness.

Growing sweet peas

If you live in a temperate climate where this plant will thrive, prepare the soil and follow the instructions on the pack to sow the seeds that will deliver fragrant sweet pea plants in midsummer. (If you live somewhere where the climate is more extreme, choose another flowering plant that you know will thrive.).

As you gently sow your sweet pea seeds and pat down the soil, think about how this plant will reward you with the heady fragrance of its blossoms if you treat it right, treat it with Kindness and take care of its needs.

When those first little spindly seedlings poke through the soil, you'll feel a nurturing protectiveness about them and before long, you'll realise something important which is that the tiny tendrils need some kind of solid support.

Handling the tendrils gently, give them support by staking them to something that will encourage their healthy growth.

What's the lesson here? We all start out a little spindly and we all need kind and loving support so that we too can thrive and send out our own 'tendrils' to explore the world.

No one is useless in this world
who lightens the burdens of another.

Charles Dickens
NOVELIST

Treat everyone with
respect and kindness.
Period.
No exceptions.

Kiana Tom
US TV HOST AND PERSONAL TRAINER

Melting Hearts

There is nothing more powerful than Kindness for melting even the most hardened of hearts and the simplest question that will show you that — just ask someone, How can I help you? What can I do?

   If they knock you back, don't take it personally.
We live in a world where Kindness has gone into hiding in many places and people may be initially suspicious of your kind-hearted intentions.

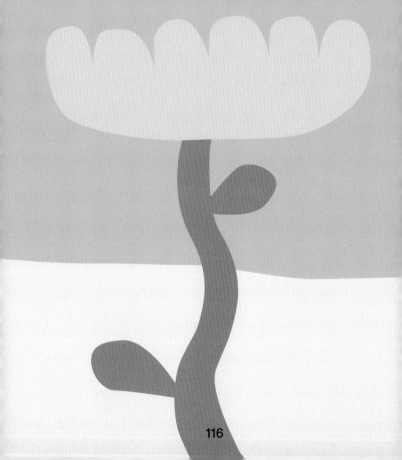

There's a revealing YouTube clip on the www.kindness.org website which tells the story of a Londoner, Joe, who decided to spend the day doing kind things for people.

The video of what happened when he went up to complete strangers to offer help went viral with more than six million Facebook views in the first 24 hours after it was posted.

But in some ways, it was a really sad indictment of how suspicious people have become of each other because most of the people he offered to help looked at him with alarm, shook their heads and walked quickly away.

If offering to help proves too intrusive for one person, try someone else. Keep going until someone is brave enough to accept your kind offer.

The Helper's High

When we do something kind for someone else, we feel good about ourselves.

Fact.

And that's thanks to chemical changes in our brain which are triggered when we do something kind.

The main hormone involved is oxytocin — sometimes called The Love Hormone.

This feel-good chemical plays a role in forming social bonds and trusting other people, creating what is known as Helper's High.

There's something about
kindness that warms our world
and makes it glow a little brighter –
as if, when we bear witness to it,
a sun rises inside of us.

Michael Winn

WWW.CHANNELKINDNESS.ORG

CHAPTER FOUR

The Currency of Kindness

Kindness comes in many forms
but is always from the heart.

It also melts hearts.

And scientists now think being
kind is encoded in our DNA!

According to scientists who reported
their findings in the journal, Proceedings
of the National Academy of Sciences, being kind,
caring, empathic and trustworthy may be an
integral part of our genetical makeup and not
a genetic accident! How good is that?

Kind words do not cost much yet they accomplish much.

Blaise Pascal
PHILOSOPHER AND WRITER

Wiccan witches and other traditions believe what you give out in life, you get back three-fold. Once you start to spread a little Kindness, you'll be astonished by how much comes straight back at you — we call this the boomerang effect!

This is not, of course, why you are working on being kind (and becoming kinder) but it's not a bad bonus. Plus, unlike Bitcoin or investing in stocks and shares, you don't need any start-up funds.

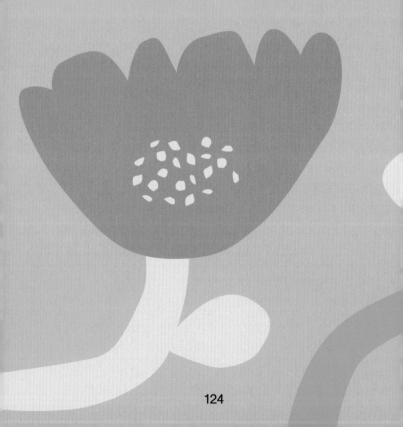

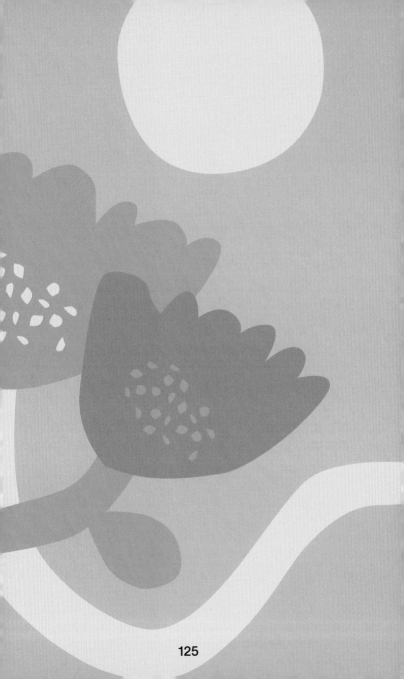

In your Kindness journal list three ways you could spend your money that would generate more Kindness in the world.
For example:

Support an animal sanctuary

Buy a Christmas gift box, for a child living in poverty in the underdeveloped world

Shop sustainably, which is being kind to the planet

Happiness is the new rich.
Inner peace is the new success.
Health is the new wealth.
Kindness is the new cool.

Syed Balkhi
AWARD-WINNING ENTREPRENEUR

Kindness has Strong Roots

The point of being kind is to be kind for its own sake, and not to expect any reward.

When you begin to practice profound and radical kindness in your life you will experience a stronger sense of your own place in the world. You will stand tall and rooted in kindness. You will have more than enough kindness to share with others, even those who pass only momentarily through your life.

The magic of being kind, for its own sake, is that anything that does come from it will be an unexpected delight and bonus in your life.

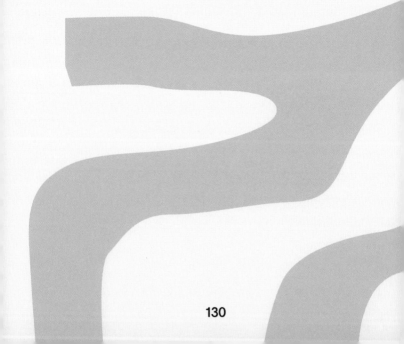

A single act
of kindness
throws out
roots in all directions,
and the roots
spring up and
make new trees

Amelia Earhart
AVIATION PIONEER

Kindness Does Not Need
to be Rationed

There's no need to be stingy with your kind deeds.

They can cost nothing and mean everything to those on the receiving end.

In fact, you can give, give, give when the heart that is guiding you is a kind one.

And when you've done that, give a little more!

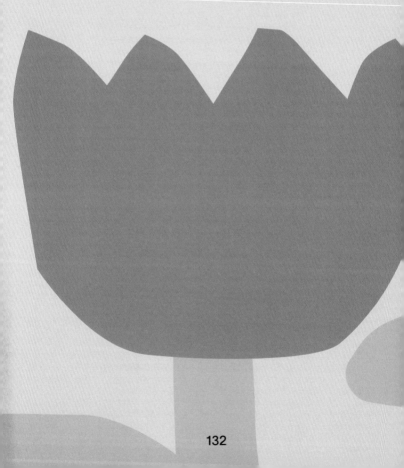

Be kind to unkind people
They need it the most.

Ashleigh Brilliant
CARTOONIST

You can always give something –
even if it is only kindness.

Anne Frank
DIARIST

No act of kindness is ever too small. The gift of kindness may start as a small ripple that over time can turn into a tidal wave affecting the lives of many.

Kevin Heath

AUSTRALIAN SPORTSMAN

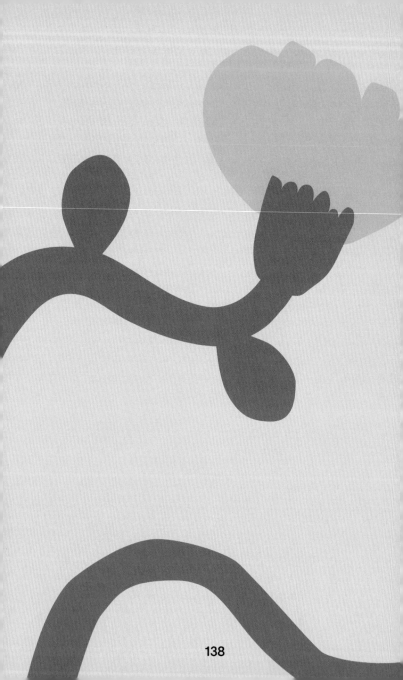

Kindness Can Change How We Think About Success

Once we begin to understand that Kindness is a currency freely available to us all to exchange and share, life begins to take on a whole new meaning.

You no longer feel rich or poor, depending on what's in your bank account.

Of course, money matters and is important for paying your way and paying your bills but it's not who you are.

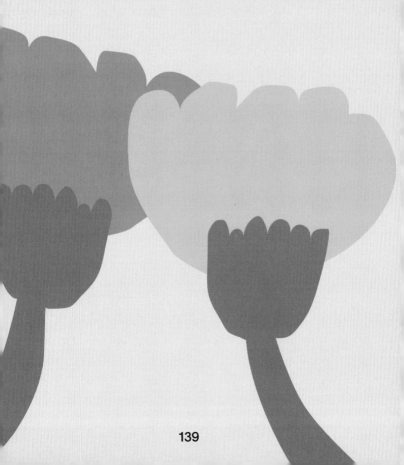

Every act of kindness is like a pebble thrown in a pond sending out ripples far beyond where the pebble entered the water. When we're caring and kind to our neighbors, our actions send rings of kindness that spread from neighbor to neighbor to neighbor.

Angela Artemis

INTUITION AND BUSINESS COACH

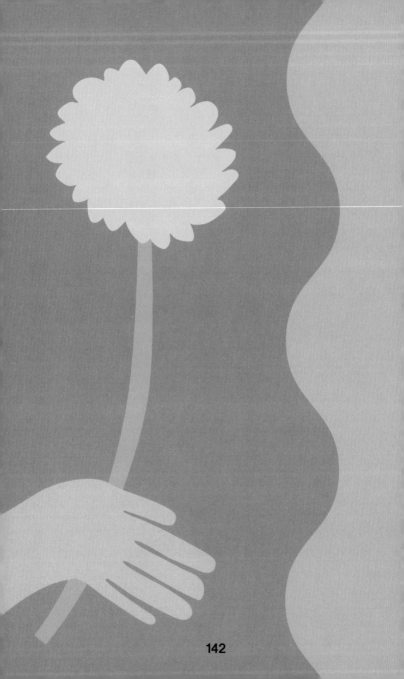

Create A Kindness Circle

You're going to love this simple but powerful exercise which, with each act of Kindness you share or exchange, sends ripples of joy and happiness out into the wider world.

Start a WhatsApp group called
The Kindness Experiment.

With Kindness as your currency of choice, you will be making it clear to people who you are and what you are all about.

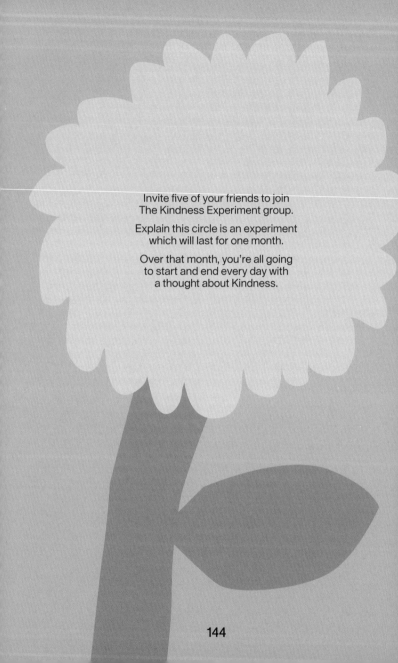

Invite five of your friends to join
The Kindness Experiment group.

Explain this circle is an experiment
which will last for one month.

Over that month, you're all going
to start and end every day with
a thought about Kindness.

144

You may share a kind deed someone has done for you or something you've done for someone else.

Enjoy these daily insights and exchanges all about Kindness and see how, when you get to the end of the month, nobody will want to leave the experiment which can now become a bona fide Kindness Circle.

EXERCISE

In your Kindness Journal write down
five new things you learned about
the friends you invited to join the
Kindness Experiment.

Write down five things you
learned about yourself.

Did the experiment
make you kinder to others?

Did you become kinder to yourself?

What's your favourite
thing about being part of
a Kindness Circle?

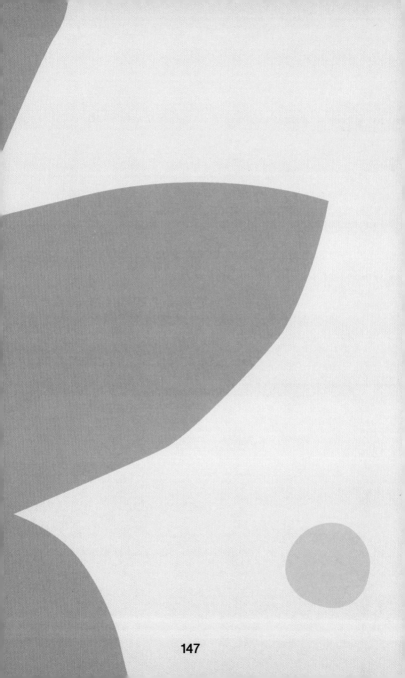

148

When we seek to discover
the best in others,
we somehow bring out
the best in ourselves.

William Arthur Ward
MOTIVATIONAL WRITER

Kindness
is free;
pass it on ...

Forget injuries, Never forget Kindness.

Confucius
CHINESE PHILOSOPHER

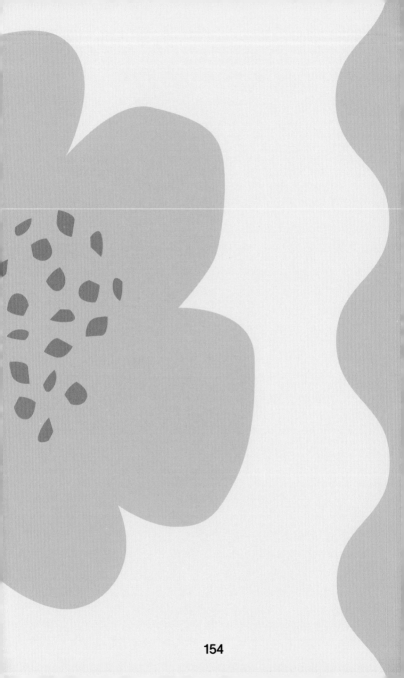

Offer a
Kindness today ...

Think about someone who would benefit from
a small act or word of Kindness right now.

This could be someone who's just lost their job
or a beloved pet or their self- confidence.

Light your Kindness candle and spend some quiet time
thinking about this person's struggle and how Kindness
will show them, however
bad things feel right now, someone cares.

As you think about this person and
their struggles, you may know just what
you can do to help.

If you don't have this lightbulb moment,
don't worry.

Contact them and ask what they need
and what you can do?

Remember, Kindness comes at
'No Charge!'

There are many different ways we can show kindness to others, and it doesn't have to be in a big way. The simplest of things may make the difference.

Catherine Pulsifer

AUTHOR

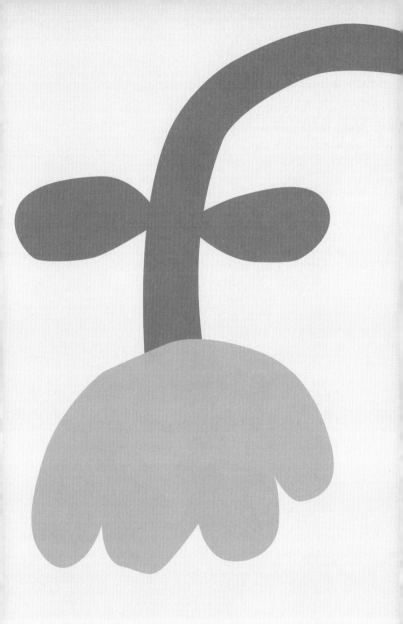

Trading in Kindness

Once we start to look at Kindness as a kind of currency, it makes sense to think about how we can easily treat it the same as any other currency and start trading in it right away.

Nobody does a kind act for someone else because they expect something back but there's no reason why you can't agree with your Kindness Circle, family, friends or work colleagues to set up a Kindness Exchange. This means doing something kind for each other every week or even every day.

You can have fun drawing up a list of kind acts and intentions and putting your name alongside those you want to deliver.

Kindness in words
creates confidence.

Kindness in thinking
creates profoundness.

Kindness in giving
creates love.

Lao Tzu
PHILOSOPHER AND FOUNDER OF TAOISM

Ideas for a Kindness Exchange

Go about these little acts of Kindness as quietly as a little mouse.Expect nothing in return but find your reward in relishing how good being kind makes you feel about yourself.

It is never too late to nourish and nurture a kind heart, at home or in the workplace and with every kind act you deliver, you will feel yourself growing taller and stronger as a kind person.

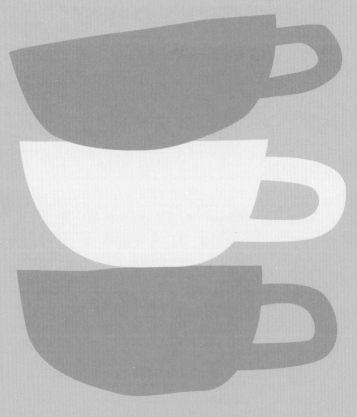

At work

Wash all the coffee cups languishing
in or near the sink, not just your own.

At home

Clean the back of the murky fridge or store
cupboard. It may not be your turn but it's
one of those jobs nobody likes doing and
everyone will appreciate the kind gesture.

At the weekend

Don't just bake one cake, bake two
and give one away with a smile.

We can't help everyone,
But everyone can help someone.

Ronald Reagan
US PRESIDENT

I've been searching
for ways to heal myself,
and I've found that kindness
is the best way.

Lady Gaga
MUSICIAN

Kindness Coins

Making your Kindness Coins

For this exercise you'll be making your own Kindness coins from whatever material you choose; this can be fabric or cardboard or even painted out-of-commission old pennies you've picked up from the second-hand store.

Once you have a pile of homemade 'coins', allocate acts of Kindness to each one.

Get the friends in your Kindness Circle to do this exercise as well and once you have a stockpile, start trading them for real.

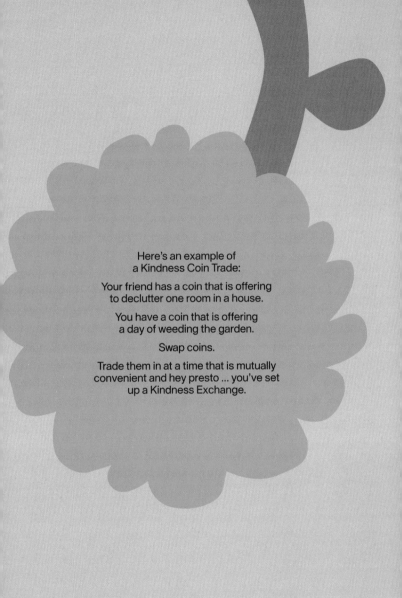

Here's an example of
a Kindness Coin Trade:

Your friend has a coin that is offering
to declutter one room in a house.

You have a coin that is offering
a day of weeding the garden.

Swap coins.

Trade them in at a time that is mutually
convenient and hey presto ... you've set
up a Kindness Exchange.

A little thought and a little
kindness are often worth more
than a great deal of money.

John Ruskin
SOCIAL THINKER

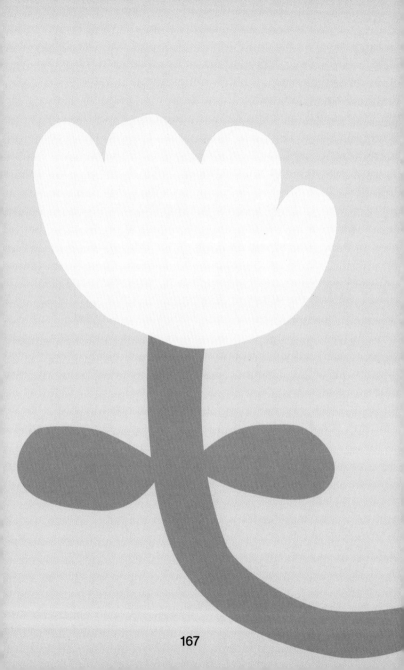

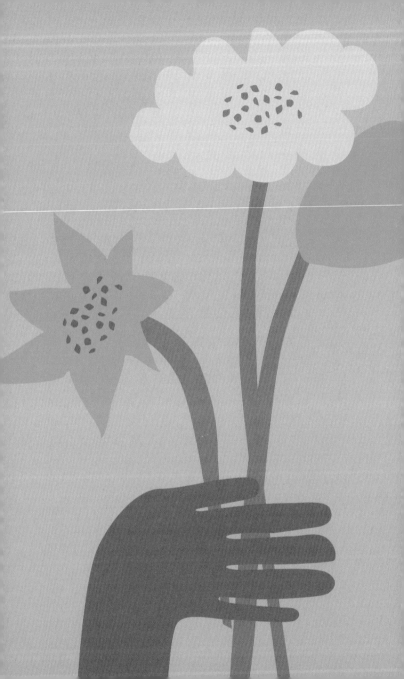

CHAPTER FIVE

Kindness Keeps Faith

A part of kindness consists of loving people more than they deserve.

Joseph Joubert
FRENCH MORALIST

As we've already seen, Kindness is not a weakness. It can take great strength to choose the path of Kindness and turn away from being mean, however justified your grievance.

Kindness is a practice; the more you do it, the better you'll get at it but don't expect to be an expert from the 'Get Go'.

Sometimes your kind gestures may backfire, be misunderstood or dismissed out of hand.

Don't give up. Get up the next day and do another kind thing for another person.

Random and Regular
Acts of Kindness

1

Hold the door open for someone
and smile as they pass through and
thank you. You'll be amazed how good
this makes them (and you) feel.

2

Pick up litter and take it home for recycling or proper
disposal. Not only does this leave the environment
a nicer place to visit than before you passed (kindly)
through, it also could prevent a wild animal choking
or otherwise injuring itself on debris someone else has
thoughtlessly discarded. place for collection,
restore it to its rightful place.

3

If you see something out of place, like a plant pot
that's blown off the neighbour's wall or a waste bin
in the wrong

4

Bake a tray cake for a nearby
care home to be shared amongst
the residents.

Notice acts of kindness offered to you from your surroundings. Someone, no matter who, is doing something thoughtful for you.

Noelia Aanulds
AUTHOR

Tenderness and Kindness
are not signs of weakness
but manifestations of strength
and resolution.

Unknown

Affirmation

I will get where I wish to be by taking
a free ride ... on a leap of faith.
Where I want to be is a world where
Kindness is the virtue we value most.

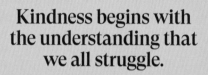

**Kindness begins with
the understanding that
we all struggle.**

Charles Glassman
LIFE COACH

Kindness itself can feel like a struggle and a step too far when we are expecting ourselves to be kind to someone who's been unkind to us.

But this is when Kindness really comes into its own.

Being kind to somebody else who's also kind is easy.

Being kind to someone who's mean is a struggle.

But it's a struggle that brings rewards — for you and for your adversary.

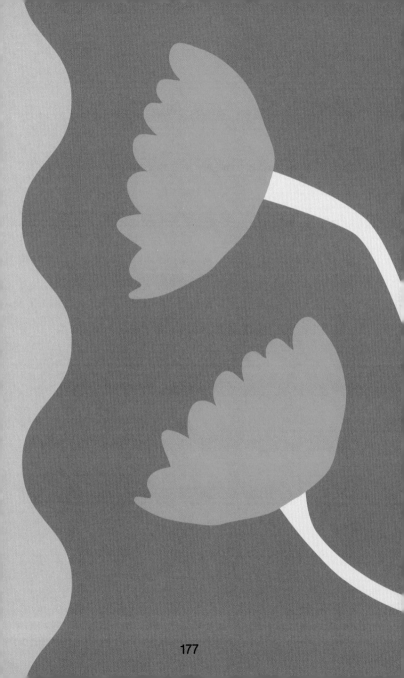

Suffering and Kindness

When things go wrong in life it's easy to get angry and upset and furious with the world.

But suffering is an inescapable part of life and one we all must learn to navigate. This is a really big part of growing as a person.

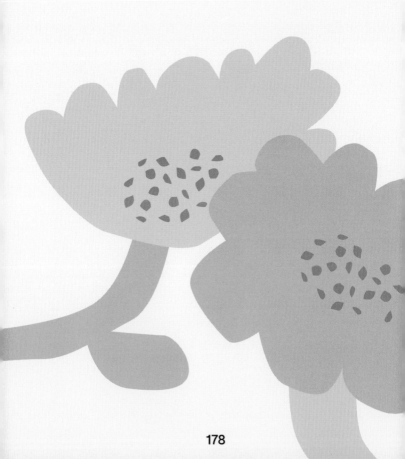

Imagine how much better you'll feel about bad things that may happen to you, if you can learn to accept your suffering with Kindness.

Kindness towards yourself
=
self-compassion

Kindness towards others,
even those who may have made
your suffering worse
=
radical compassion

Be kind, for everyone you meet is fighting a harder battle.

Ian Maclaren
AUTHOR

Next time somebody says or does something mean towards you, stop for a second or two and think about this...

Anyone you meet could be fighting some kind of private battle you know nothing about.

For some, this battle will be harder than any struggle you've ever had or can imagine.

Keep this in your mind and it will help you keep faith with Kindness.

You won't even want to be unkind.

You'll want to be kind towards them, no matter what they have said or done to hurt you.

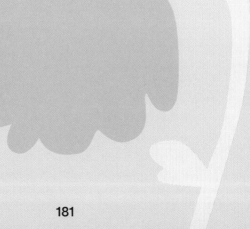

Who's the Lucky One?

In my work as a Real Life writer, I am often asked to interview people who have survived the most harrowing of times.

This is always, always my favourite type of work and there's a reason I find it so rewarding.

Whenever I talk to people who are telling a part of their life story, often the most challenging part, I am struck by how often they tell me they are 'Lucky' or 'Blessed.'

What on earth are they talking about?

How can having your health, your relationship, your home or anything else you really love ripped out from under your feet leave you feeling like 'The Lucky One?'

Of course, nobody feels 'lucky' when bad things happen but what people tell me, again and again, is that once they've survived one of life's big challenges, they are not the same person anymore.

They have become older.
And wiser.
And ... you've guessed it ...
KINDER!

They no longer sweat the small stuff —
life's too short for agitation.

They've no interest in 'dog-eat dog' — they now know
if you help raise others up, you raise yourself up too.

They've learned life really is precious and want to
share this revelation with everyone they meet.

They've learned the value of Kindness — and have
signed up to sharing that currency from now on.

One day, in retrospect,
the years of struggle will strike
you as the most beautiful.

Sigmund Freud
PSYCHOANALYST

Why Does Going Through Something Bad Make You a Kinder Person?

I'm not going to answer this question for you —
you are!

In your Kindness Journal, write about a time when something really bad happened to you and somebody else made you feel better about it, or yourself, by saying or doing something kind.

Imagine you are telling this scene
as a story to someone else.

Tell your listener how someone's unexpected
Kindness made you feel when life was bad?

Tell your listener what this experience taught
you about the importance of Kindness in the
'Bad Times'.

I have learnt silence from
the talkative, toleration from the
intolerant, and kindness from
the unkind; yet strange, I am
ungrateful to these teachers.

Khalil Gibran

POET

Affirmation

Sometimes, Kindness is just about choosing to bite your tongue!

However hard that may feel ...

And if you want to learn how to do that, go and take a look at Rain Dove's Instagram pages.

Rain Dove is an American gender non-conforming model and activist but above and beyond all this, Rain Dove has mastered the art of slaying people with Kindness.

Representing 'human' in everything they say, think and do — Kindness lies at the very heart of their actions even in the face of the most hurtful trolling.

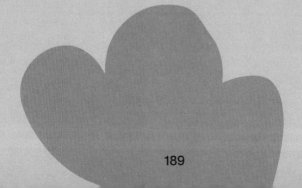

Kindness Heals

Another reason to keep faith with Kindness is that Kindness is a very powerful force for healing.

Science shows that delivering health care with Kindness leads to faster healing.

It also reduces pain, boosts immune function, lowers blood pressure and decreases anxiety.

The words of kindness are more healing to a drooping heart than balm or honey.

Sarah Fielding

AUTHOR

A soul without Kindness
Is like a garden without
plants or flowers

Debasish Mirdha
NEUROLOGIST AND PHILOSOPHER

Kindness Rituals

You don't need to buy anything or go anywhere to introduce Kindness rituals into your everyday life.

You already have the most important thing you'll need — a kind and caring heart!

A ritual can be as simple or as complex as you like but the truth is, you can turn any everyday activity into a meaningful ritual and one that you dedicate to Kindness.

Turn these everyday activities, or others, into a Kindness ritual. Approach things with a kind heart and notice the difference that makes to how you feel about what you're doing, and the end results.

Water your house plants

Talk softly to them and think about
being kind to them.

Walk your dog (or someone else's)

Use gentle tones to guide the animal who trusts
you to look out for it. Notice everything about this
animal; does it need food or water? A rest? Some
playtime? Trust that your kind heart will alert you
to what it needs.

Clean the bathroom

Approach this household chore in a spirit of
Kindness and you'll be amazed how much more
you enjoy the task. Need to scrub the shower tiles?
Do it with a kindly intent and enjoy every second
of restoring them to their former glory.

Unconditional love flows through specific channels of respect, integrity, purpose, meaning, value, response-ability, forgiveness, kindness, and compassion — and these form the foundation of our new, naturally ethical lives.

Loch Kelly

MEDITATION TEACHER

Kindness Mantra

To keep Kindness as your creed, repeat this sacred utterance out loud or in your head. You can also write your own.

I believe in Kindness
I will seek out Kindness
I can offer Kindness
Kindness is my creed

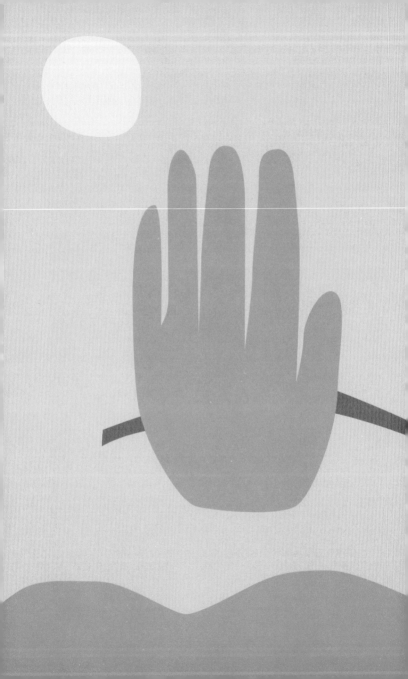

CHAPTER SIX

Ahimsa — Loving Kindness

Ahimsa is the ancient Sanskrit word yoga masters use to describe the dedicated practice of Loving Kindness which really is 'a thing!'

So let's embrace Loving Kindness and make it part of our daily Kindness practice.

A Little Yoga ....

To get started, we need to practice those simple yoga postures (asanas) that bring our attention back, again and again, to the heart chakra (our energy centre) and which remind us there's both a physical and mental strength to be found in making Loving Kindness (ahimsa) our mantra and our daily practice.

A Lot of Kindness ...

Once we've mastered these yoga postures (asanas); we can start to learn the breathing practices (pranayama) that also encourage Loving Kindness (ahimsa) in our daily lives.

We'll then learn the symbolic hand positions (mudra) we hold during meditation and easy chants (mantra) that will help us stay kind.

Yoga asanas that encourage Kindness are:

The Camel

The Bow

The Warrior

The Pose of the Child

Let's try each posture and see how it feels and by doing so, encourage our heart chakra to open even wider and fully embrace Loving Kindness.

Don't worry if you've never done yoga before. This is not a competition, with yourself or anyone else. I'll guide you very gently through each posture, but always just do whatever feels most comfortable for you.

It's your body — so listen to it and treat it with Kindness!

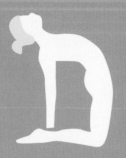

The Camel

By releasing tension in the shoulders and the back, this asana works to open up the chest increase your heart energy.

How to

1. Kneel on your mat and gently raise your body so you are 'standing' on your knees with your arms at your sides.
2. Slowly lean backwards and take hold of your legs (one in each hand) as close to the ankle as you can. DO NOT STRAIN TO DO THIS.
3. Push your tummy out and forward and let your head fall back as far as feels comfortable.
4. Hold this posture for a few seconds. Relax the back and then release.

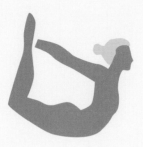

The Bow

Most people simply forget the heart is a muscle, but this posture fully acknowledges that it is and works to tone the heart and get the breath flowing nicely.

We'll try the easy version which will also help relieve stiffness in the back — something which can be a sign of 'hanging on' to the tried and tested, and feeling nervous about finding new ways in life.

How to

1. Lie flat on your tummy on your mat with your legs out straight, feet together and your arms at your side

2. Bend your knees and bring your heels in towards your bottom.

3. Take hold of both ankles, one in each hand, and put your chin on the mat.

4. Now, breathe in and focus on pushing your feet away from the body which will also lift your head from the mat.

5. Hold for a second or so as you exhale and bring the body back down to lying on the mat

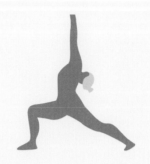

The Warrior

Use the Warrior pose to reach for a kinder version
of yourself.

How to

1. 1. Stand on your mat facing forward, arms at your side and
   feet together.
2. Put your hands on your hips to help you balance and step
   forward with your right foot.
3. Bend your right knee and slightly turn your back foot (the left
   foot) so it runs sideways across your mat. Your right foot will
   be facing forward so you've created a kind of triangle with
   your body.
4. Take a deep breath in through the nose, put the palms of
   your hands together in a prayer posture and lift your arms
   above your head, as high as you can.
5. Keep your arms touching your ears and reach, reach, reach
   for the stars — be the kindest version of you that you can be.
6. When it feels right, come back to standing on your mat.

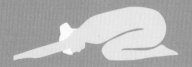

The Pose of the Child

This is one of the most gentle and peaceful poses you can do. Think about its name — the pose of the child. Think about the softness of very young children before they've had a chance to develop hard edges. This pose is all about Loving Kindness and softness.

How to

1. Kneel and gently lay your forehead on the mat.
2. Allow both arms to relax, one each side of the body with your palms facing up to the ceiling.
3. In this folded position, breathe slowly in, to a count of five.
4. Hold the breath for a count of five.
5. Exhale to a count of at least five, or longer if you can.
6. Repeat this cycle a few more times. You won't want to stop and leave this pose!

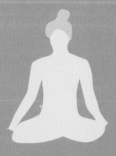

Mudra – The Lotus

This beautiful flower has its roots in the murkiest of waters, so the Lotus mudra reminds us that out of the dark comes the light.

How to

1. Sit comfortably on your mat, cross-legged, in lotus position (if that's comfortable for you) or propped up on a cushion. Whatever your body likes.

2. Close your eyes, start counting your breaths (in to five, hold for five, out for five or more) and now gently place your hands, palms together, over your heart centre, touching your thumbs and little fingers together.

3. The rest of your fingers will naturally open out like a lotus flower opening towards the sun.

4. Keep to the slow rhythm of breathing. Meditate in this position for as long as you like, thinking about Kindness and Compassion.

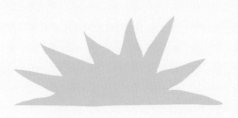

Pranayama

Pranayama is the name given to special yogic breathing practices. Once we've mastered these we will be:

Breathing for Kindness

Breathing for Peace

Breathing for Happiness

Breathing for Joy

The Humming Bee Breath

You'll feel silly the first few times you try this, but it's brilliant for calming the mind and great fun (once you get over your shyness). It may also make you feel so grateful for the work of the humble bee, without which we'd struggle to pollinate the crops we eat.

How to

1. Sit or kneel comfortably on your yoga mat and close your eyes.
2. Imagine you are a little worker bee buzzing around doing everything in your power to help your hive survive.
3. Breathe in slowly through your nose and as you breathe out, allow your vocal cords to hum or vibrate to make the buzzing noise of a bee. The more you practice this, the better you'll become at it.
4. Eventually, you can also' buzz' as you breath in, although this is harder. The sound you make might even be more screechy than buzzy at first, but eventually, you'll get the hang of it.

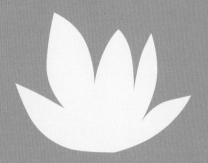

Mantra – The Buddhist Mettist prayer

Simple but deeply profound, this prayer starts by blessing yourself and gradually expands outwards until you are sending kind and loving intensions for the entire world and all beings, including anyone you don't even like!

Here are the words of this
beautiful Kindness prayer that
you will be saying out loud or
in your mind:

My heart fills with Loving Kindness. I love myself. May I be happy.
May I be well. May I be peaceful. May I be free.

May all beings in my vicinity be happy. May they be well.
May they be peaceful. May they be free.

May all beings in my city be happy. May they be well.
May they be peaceful. May they be free.

May all beings in my community be happy. May they be well.
May they be peaceful. May they be free.

May all beings in my country be happy. May they be well.
May they be peaceful. May they be free.

May all beings on my continent be happy. May they be well.
May they be peaceful. May they be free.

May all beings in my hemisphere be happy. May they be well.
May they be peaceful. May they be free.

May all beings on planet Earth be happy. May they be well.
May they be peaceful. May they be free.

May my parents be happy. May they be well.
May they be peaceful. May they be free.

May all my friends be happy. May they be well.
May they be peaceful. May they be free.

May all my enemies be happy. May they be well.
May they be peaceful. May they be free.

May all beings in the Universe be happy. May they be well.
May they be peaceful. May they be free.

If I have hurt anyone, knowingly or unknowingly
in thought, word or deed, I ask for their forgiveness.

If anyone has hurt me, knowingly or unknowingly
in thought, word or deed, I extend my forgiveness.

May all beings everywhere, whether near or far,
whether known to me or unknown, be happy.
May they be well. May they be peaceful.
May they be free.

In these last few pages, we'll briefly sum up what we've learned about Kindness with a capital 'K'; remind ourselves why it's so important to make Kindness central to all our life choices and see again how, happily, the more we choose Kindness the kinder and kinder we become.

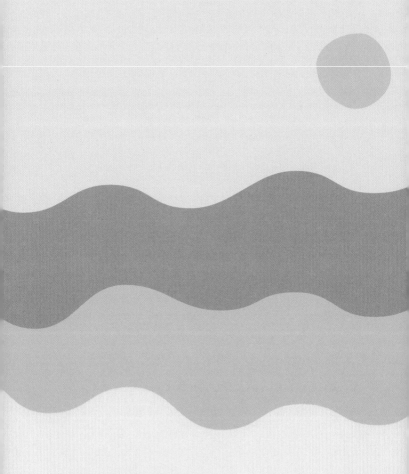

K

is for ...

**Keeping the powerful flame
of Kindness burning in our
very core.**

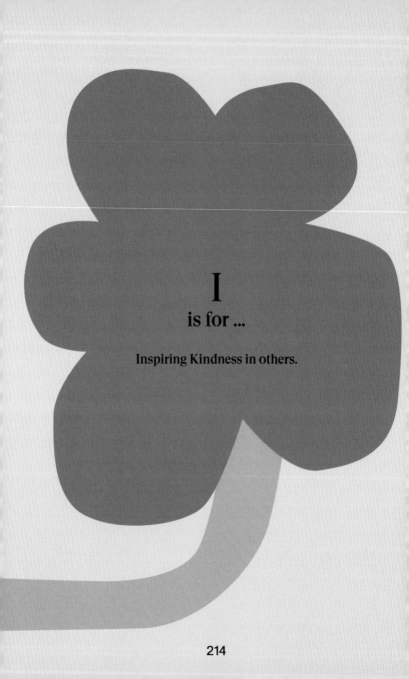

I

is for ...

Inspiring Kindness in others.

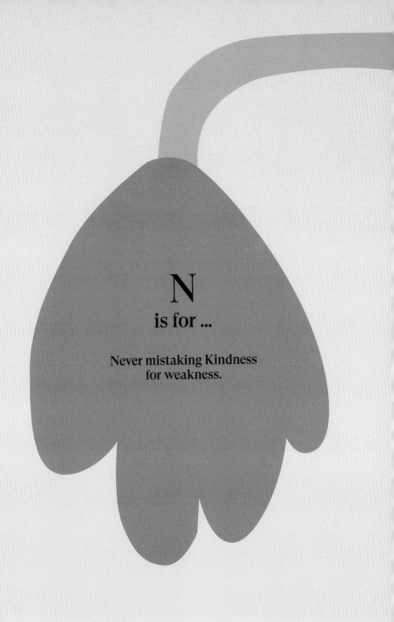

N
is for ...

Never mistaking Kindness
for weakness.

D
is for ...

Doing our best to sprinkle
Kindness everywhere we go and
over everything we do.

216

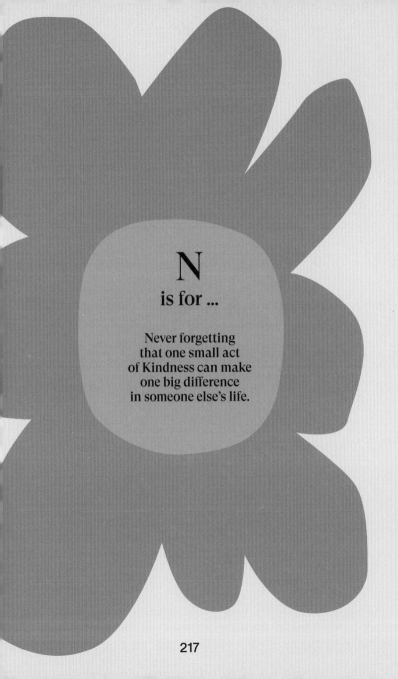

N
is for ...

Never forgetting
that one small act
of Kindness can make
one big difference
in someone else's life.

E

is for ...

**Engaging with Kindness
every chance we get and exploring
all the ways we can be kind and kinder
to ourselves and each other.**

S

is for ...

**Sharing everything we've learned
about Kindness in this little book
with everyone we meet.**

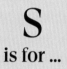

S

is for ...

Shaping and sharing a new
world view – one that is built
on Kindness.

A Final Thought ...

Kindness sticks!

Throughout the writing of this book, I've had, not surprisingly, Kindness foremost in my mind. And that got me to thinking about people I've met who really do live daily lives of Kindness —
often without even realising they do and certainly never once boasting that they do!

When the Coronavirus Pandemic struck in early 2020, I volunteered for a time — to help deliver shopping and meals — with a group of people based in Crewkerne in South Somerset in the UK who for me, personified Kindness in everything they said and did.

They were all shining examples of what it means to live out a life dedicated to service and Kindness. I found it inspiring to be among them.

Here they all are:

Paul, Rob, Mike, Maggie, Simon, Jackie and Steve.

'The Crewkerne Kindness Crew.'

Acknowledgements

With thanks to my publisher, Kate Pollard, for steering her vision of a book that will inspire Kindness in all who read it my way. And to our editor, Jo Hanks, for her attention to diversity and detail, and the design team at Evi O. Studio.

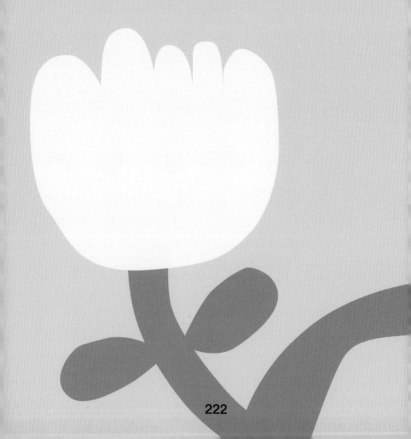

About the Author

Susan Elizabeth Clark is a self-help writer who specialises in shining a light on those topics that can help people overcome their challenges to live their best lives. She has studied esoteric traditions and yoga in both India and the UK. Susan lives in Yorkshire.

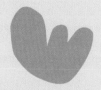

Published by OH Editions
20 Mortimer Street
London W1T 3JW

Design © 2021 OH Editions

ISBN 978-1-914317-01-9

Text © Susan Elizabeth Clark
Editorial: Jo Hanks
Design and illustrations: Evi-O.Studio | Kait Polkinghorne & Susan Le
Production: Rachel Burgess

A CIP catalogue record for this book is available
from the British Library

Printed and bound in China.

10 9 8 7 6 5 4 3 2 1